The Longest *Goodbye*

A Guided Journal for Individuals
Caring for Their Loved One With Dementia

Kellie Vanella

Copyright © 2023 Kellie Vanella

All rights reserved. No part of this book may be reproduced in any form without permission from the author or publisher, except as permitted by U.S. copyright law.

To request permission, contact
unmaskautism@gmail.com

ISBN: 979-8-9888757-1-0
Second Edition

Published by Unmask Publishing House
Virginia Beach, VA
UnmaskAutism.com

This
Journal
belongs to:

_____

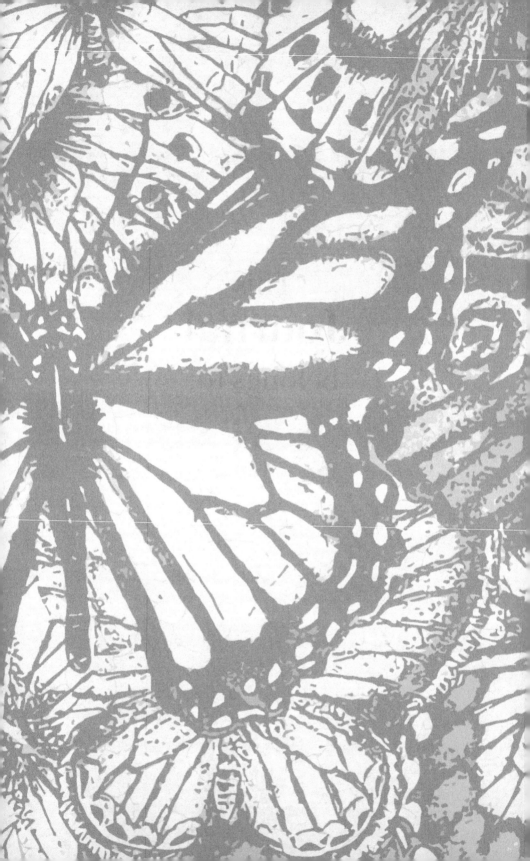

Introduction

Welcome to "The Longest Goodbye: A Guided Journal for Individuals Caring for Their Loved One With Dementia." Caring for a loved one with dementia is a journey filled with deep love and enormous hardships. This journal grew from my experience caring for my mother as she battled Frontotemporal Dementia. This journal aims to give individuals on a similar path a place to explore many feelings regarding the difficulties of caring for a loved one with dementia.

Caring for someone with dementia requires a great deal of patience, compassion, and strength. This role often feels lonely and underappreciated, as the loved one receiving care necessitates near-constant attention. However, it is crucial to remember that your well-being and emotional health as a caregiver are equally important.

You will explore many aspects of caring for yourself as you navigate the complicated aspects of your caregiving journey in this journal full of thoughtfully curated, thought-provoking prompts. Each section will cover a specific topic essential for your well-being and growth as a caregiver.

Beginning with identifying potential signs of caregiver burnout, this journal acknowledges the physical, mental, and emotional demands placed on caretakers. It emphasizes the critical need to recognize when you are reaching your limits. Knowing the signs and symptoms of burnout allows you to prevent it and ensure you take care of yourself proactively.

Following that, you will consider how meditation, mindfulness practices, and prayer can assist you in your caregiving journey. These practices can provide solace, rejuvenation, and a sense of inner peace amidst the ever-changing chaos of caregiving. They are effective instruments for finding moments of solitude that will recharge your spirit.

One of the most challenging aspects of caring for someone with dementia is navigating their behaviors. It's easy to take these actions personally, but it's critical not to. You will investigate how changing your thoughts and responses might alter your perspective and assist you in navigating challenging situations with grace and compassion. This will allow you to maintain your bond with your loved one during your difficult journey together.

Maintaining connections and asking for help are essential aspects of caregiving. Therefore, the need to seek assistance for yourself, whether through friends, family, or support groups, is emphasized in this journal. You will also consider how maintaining relationships with others can give you a sense of community and understanding.

Physical health is critical for maintaining the energy and stamina needed for caregiving. You will look into emphasizing self-care habits like regular exercise and adequate rest. You can better meet caregiving responsibilities if you prioritize your well-being.

This journal will also encourage you to schedule regular breaks for yourself. You will discuss how, amidst caregiving responsibilities, you might create moments of rest and self-renewal despite the time and resource restraints standard with caretaking roles.

Grief is an unavoidable component of the caring-giving experience. As you watch your loved ones' abilities deteriorate, you must begin processing your grief. As you negotiate the complicated emotions that surface during this process, this journal will provide an outlet to process the feelings that arise.

Finally, in "The Longest Goodbye," you will learn how to treasure the new memories you make with your loved one throughout your caregiving journey. Despite the difficulties, you will recognize moments of joy, connection, and love that should be celebrated. You will find satisfaction and gratitude in your caregiving journey when you embrace these moments that will become lifelong memories.

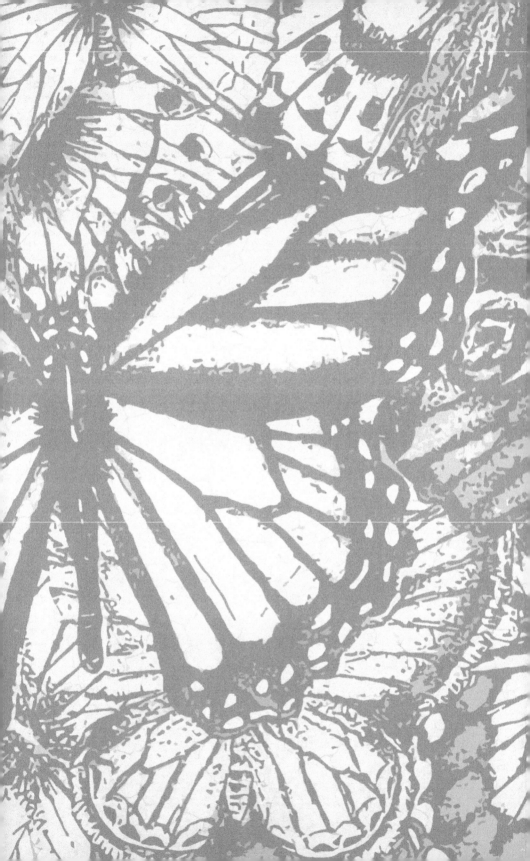

Recognizing Caretaker Burnout

Caring for someone with dementia is a never-ending challenge. As a caregiver, you must be aware of the indications of burnout since neglecting your well-being might jeopardize the quality of care you provide. In this journal section, you will investigate ways to minimize or mitigate caregiver burnout. Please consider your thoughts and feelings as you navigate this critical issue.

Physical exhaustion is one of the most apparent indications of burnout. Do you feel exhausted no matter how much sleep you get? Take note of any physical symptoms you may be having, such as headaches, muscle tightness, or sleeping difficulties. Recognizing these signs can assist you in addressing your needs and managing your care.

Another significant component of burnout is emotional exhaustion. Are you feeling overwhelmed, angry, or emotionally depleted? Do you find yourself having frequent mood swings or feeling depressed all of the time? Recognize and validate your emotions since they are essential to your general well-being. Understanding your emotional state is the first step toward finding successful coping methods.

Have you been ignoring your own needs? Caregivers frequently put their loved one's needs ahead of their own, but it's critical to remember that self-care is not selfish. Consider whether you are eating healthily, getting enough exercise, and participating in things that bring you joy. Remember that caring for yourself is as important as caring for others.

Caregiving is frequently associated with social isolation. Is it challenging for you to maintain social contacts outside of your caretaker role? Have you stopped participating in activities or neglected your relationships with friends and family? Recognize the value of support networks and investigate strategies to strengthen your social connections while caring for your loved one.

Recognizing burnout symptoms is the first step toward managing it. By identifying these warning signs, you can take action to safeguard your health and maintain your capacity to care for your loved one. This section will explore how you can implement strategies and techniques to prevent and manage caregiver burnout effectively. Remember that addressing your health is critical for you and your loved one.

Reflect on your journey as a caretaker so far. What are some of the challenges you have faced in caring for your loved one with dementia?

How has being a caretaker impacted your emotional well-being?
Describe some of the emotions you have experienced and how they
have influenced your overall mental health.

Explore the concept of burnout. How would you define burnout as a caretaker? Have you ever experienced burnout? If so, what were the signs and symptoms you noticed?

Think about the physical toll of caregiving. How has it affected your own physical health? Consider any changes you may have noticed in your sleeping patterns, energy levels, or overall physical stamina.

Consider the guilt and self-judgment that may arise as a caretaker. Have you ever felt guilty for taking time for yourself or prioritizing your own needs? How can you work towards letting go of these feelings?

Imagine a day without caregiving responsibilities. How would you choose to spend that day? What activities or hobbies bring you joy and rejuvenation?

Describe your dreams and aspirations beyond caregiving. What are some goals or dreams you have for your own life? How can you work towards incorporating these aspirations into your current role as a caretaker?

Explore the role of self-compassion in preventing and managing caretaker burnout. How can you cultivate self-compassion and practice kindness towards yourself during challenging moments?

Consider the importance of self-reflection and self-awareness as a caretaker. How can you become more attuned to your own needs and emotions in order to prevent or recover from burnout?

Imagine the ideal support system for a caretaker. What resources or assistance would be most helpful for you? How can you work towards creating or accessing these supports?

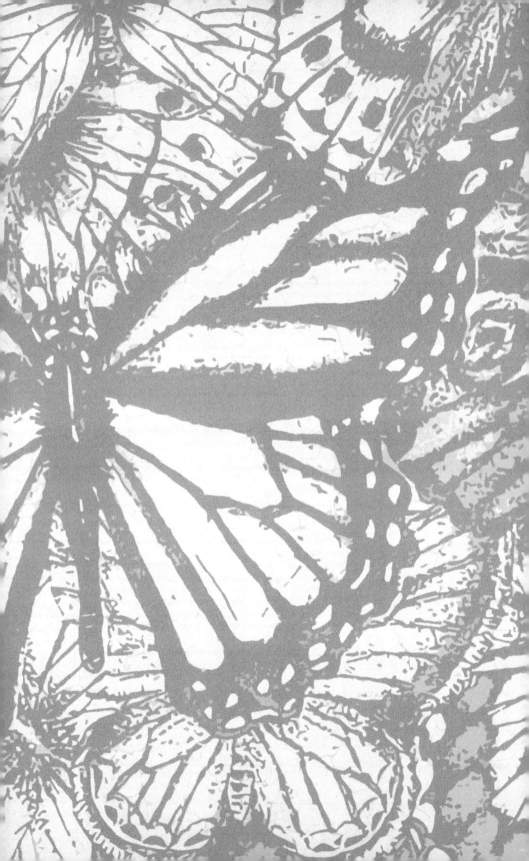

Practicing Meditation, Mindfulness Activities, and Prayer

It is easy to become overwhelmed by the ongoing demands and problems of caring for someone with dementia. Finding calm and tranquillity amid turmoil is critical for your health. In this journal section, you will learn about the benefits of meditation, mindfulness, and prayer to restore balance in your life. Meditation is a highly effective practice for relaxation and self-reflection. Do you already meditate as part of your everyday routine? If not, have you thought about it? Spend a few moments sitting quietly, concentrating on your breathing, and allowing your mind to rest. Without passing judgment, take note of any thoughts or feelings that come. Meditation daily can help reduce stress, increase mental clarity, and promote inner serenity.

Mindfulness activities are also suitable for carers' well-being. Activities like strolling in nature, journaling, or doing yoga can help you be present in the moment and create a sense of gratitude amid hardship. You will find relief from caregiving's stresses and uncertainties if you focus on the present. Allow yourself the time and space to thoroughly immerse yourself in these activities, savoring the simple pleasures they bring.

Prayer brings peace and strength to individuals who find assurance in their spirituality. Whether through organized religious practices or personal reflections, prayer grounds you and provides solace amid your most challenging moments as a caretaker. Take a few moments to consider your spiritual beliefs and how spiritual practices like prayer can help you on your caring-taking journey. Remember that meditation, mindfulness, and prayer are about finding moments of solitude and self-care to recharge your batteries and nourish your spirit. You can better care for your loved one and negotiate caregiving obstacles with resilience and grace if you invest in your well-being.

Focus on your breath as it enters and leaves your body, allowing it to anchor you in the present moment. Write about any moments of calm or clarity you experienced during the meditation and how you can bring those moments into your caregiving interactions.

Take a slow, mindful walk with your loved one, paying attention to the sights, sounds, and sensations around you. Describe any observations or connections you made during the walk that brought you closer to your loved one or helped you see the world from their perspective.

Imagine a calm, peaceful place and visualize yourself and your loved one in that setting. Describe the details of this visualization and reflect on how it brings you a sense of peace or respite from the difficulties of caregiving.

Allow yourself to fully experience and release any emotions that may arise during your caregiving journey. Write about the emotions that surfaced during the meditation and how acknowledging and processing them can contribute to your overall well-being and resilience as a caregiver.

Say a prayer of surrender, acknowledging that there are limitations to what you can control and asking for guidance and strength. Explore your feelings of surrender and reflect on how this practice helps you release any burdens or expectations you may be carrying.

Engage in activities that nurture your own well-being and replenish your energy, such as taking a warm bath, reading a book, or practicing a hobby. Write about how practicing mindful self-care positively impacts your caregiving role and allows you to show up more fully for your loved one.

Practice active listening when communicating with your loved one, fully focusing on their words, tone, and body language. Write about any new discoveries or deeper understanding you gained from practicing mindful listening and how it can improve your communication and connection.

Say a prayer of compassion and understanding for your loved one, recognizing their struggles and asking for their peace and comfort. Write about the emotions and insights that surfaced during the prayer and how it can enhance your empathy and patience in your caregiving role.

49

Reflect on the concept of acceptance in relation to caregiving, recognizing that there are limitations and changes that are beyond your control. Explore your feelings and thoughts on acceptance and how it can help you find peace and resilience in your caregiving journey.

Go for a walk outdoors and actively seek out things to be grateful for, such as the beauty of nature or acts of kindness from others. Describe the moments of gratitude that emerged during the walk and how this practice can shift your perspective and bring more positivity into your caregiving experience.

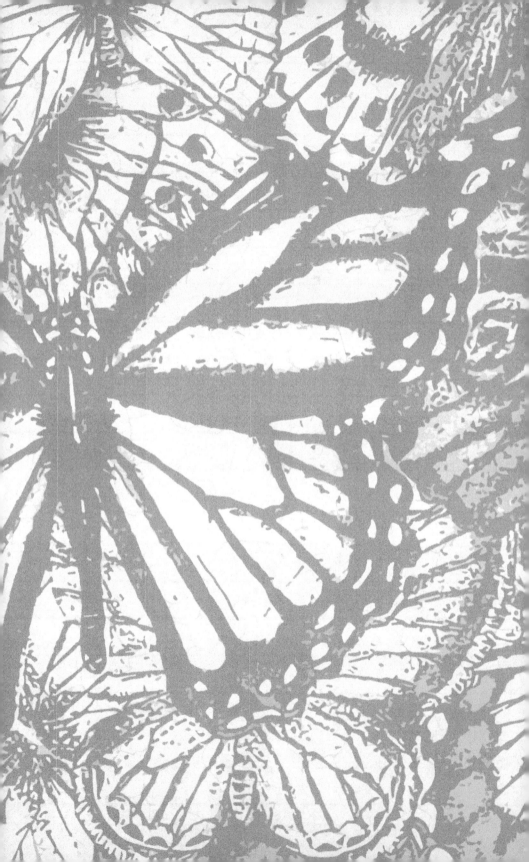

Not Taking Behaviors Personally

Caring for someone with dementia can be emotionally draining, especially when dealing with complex behaviors or disorientation. It is critical to remember not to take these behaviors personally. In this journal section, you will begin establishing your techniques to assist you in managing the complicated behaviors you face with empathy and understanding.

Dementia impairs a person's cognitive abilities, memory, and reality perception. As a result, individuals may exhibit out-of-character or even harmful actions. This can include angry and frustrated expressions such as rude remarks or physical aggressiveness toward their caregiver. Remember that these behaviors do not reflect their genuine personality or feelings toward you.

When confronted with challenging actions, remember that your loved one is experiencing their distinct reality and may struggle to convey their needs or emotions adequately. Take a step back and try to figure out what's causing their behavior. Are they in pain or afraid? Considering the potential cause may allow you to respond with patience rather than reacting out of frustration or hurt.

Journaling can be an effective method for processing and managing the various emotions that arise as a caregiver. Consider occasions when your loved one's dementia-related behaviors have negatively impacted you. Examine your feelings and thoughts about these situations. Consider how you may reframe your perspective so you do not take these behaviors personally. Consider skills or self-care routines to help you stay grounded amid these difficult behaviors. Remember that caring for someone with dementia requires tremendous strength and compassion. You can approach your caregiving position with greater understanding and empathy if you remind yourself not to take their actions personally. As you negotiate the complications of dementia caregiving with grace and resilience, embrace the journey of self-reflection and growth.

Describe a recent challenging behavior exhibited by your loved one with dementia. How did you initially react to it?

57

Reflect on a time when you took a dementia behavior personally. How did it affect your emotional well-being and relationship with your loved one?

How can you remind yourself that dementia behaviors are not a reflection of your loved one's true self?

What strategies can you employ to cultivate empathy and understanding towards your loved one's behaviors, even when challenging or frustrating?

Write a letter to yourself, reminding you not to take dementia behaviors personally. What affirmations or reminders can you include to help shift your perspective?

Share a story or experience where you were able to respond to a very challenging dementia behavior with patience, love, and understanding. How did it impact your relationship with your loved one?

Explore the concept of separating the person from the disease. How can you remind yourself that your loved one's behaviors are not a reflection of their true self, but rather a manifestation of their dementia?

Write about a specific strategy or coping mechanism you have found effective in reminding yourself not to take dementia behaviors personally. How does this strategy help you maintain your emotional well-being as a caregiver?

71

Consider the impact of self-care on your ability to not take dementia behaviors personally. How does prioritizing your own well-being help you approach these behaviors with more empathy and understanding?

Consider seeking support from other caregivers who can relate to your experiences. Reflect on the benefits of sharing your challenges and learning from others who have faced similar situations.

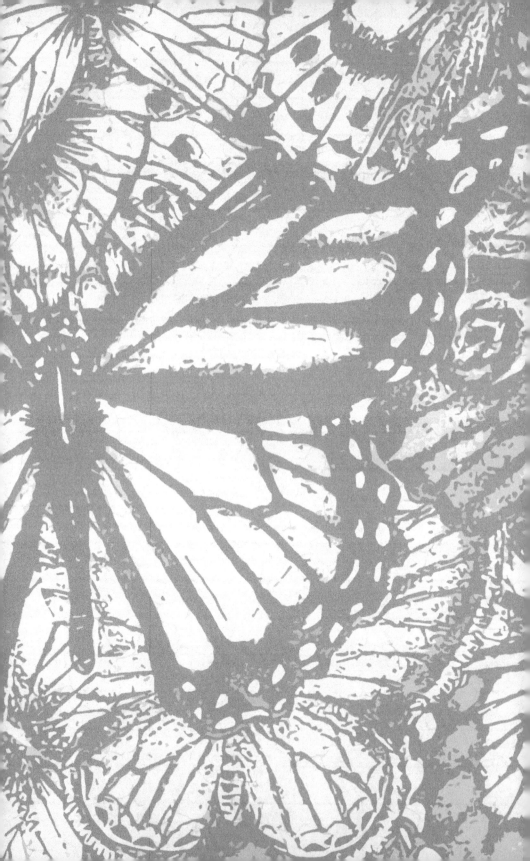

Modifying Your Thoughts and Adapting Your Responses

Caring for a loved one with dementia is a journey that necessitates ongoing adaptation and flexibility. As a caregiver, you may face various emotional and functional challenges as you negotiate the ever-evolving circumstances of dementia. In this journal section, you will learn how to adjust your thoughts and adapt your responses as a caretaker, allowing you to understand better and meet your loved one's unique needs.

As previously noted, dementia causes various cognitive and behavioral changes that can be challenging to understand and navigate. It is critical to note that how you think about and respond to these problems can significantly impact your well-being and the quality of care you deliver. Modifying your thoughts entails challenging preconceived notions, reframing negative views, and adopting a more empathic and caring attitude toward the circumstances of your loved one.

Remember that the dementia care journey is not static, necessitating continual adaptation and learning. Changing your responses is synonymous with changing your thoughts. To better connect with and assist your loved one, you must be open to learning, growing, and adapting your approach. Every person with dementia is different; what works for one person might not work for another. You can adjust your care to your loved one's needs, preferences, and capabilities by modifying your thoughts and adapting your responses.

Reflect on a recent negative thought or assumption you have had about your caregiving role. How could you reframe that thought to be more adaptive and empowering?

_____

_____

_____

_____

_____

_____

_____

_____

_____

_____

_____

_____

_____

_____

_____

What are some common negative thought patterns that arise during caregiving? How can you consciously challenge and modify these thoughts?

How can you practice self-compassion and offer yourself grace during challenging moments as a caregiver?

Identify a specific situation where you tend to have automatic negative thoughts. Brainstorm adaptive responses that can help you reframe those thoughts more positively and constructively.

How can you cultivate resilience and flexibility in your thinking to better adapt to the ever-changing nature of dementia caregiving?

Describe a time when you successfully modified your thoughts and responses to a challenging situation. How did it impact your overall well-being and the caregiving experience?

Write about a time when you struggled with accepting the reality of your loved one's condition and how it impacted your ability to adapt your responses. How can you modify your thoughts and embrace acceptance to better support both yourself and your loved one?

Explore the concept of empathy and it's role in modifying your thoughts and responses when caring for someone with dementia. How can you cultivate empathy and use it to better understand and connect with your loved one?

Reflect on a situation where you found yourself feeling guilty or inadequate as a caregiver. How can you modify your thoughts and practice self-compassion to let go of these negative emotions and continue providing care with love and understanding?

Write about a specific communication challenge you've encountered while caring for your loved one with dementia. How can you modify your thoughts and adapt your communication style to better connect and engage with them?

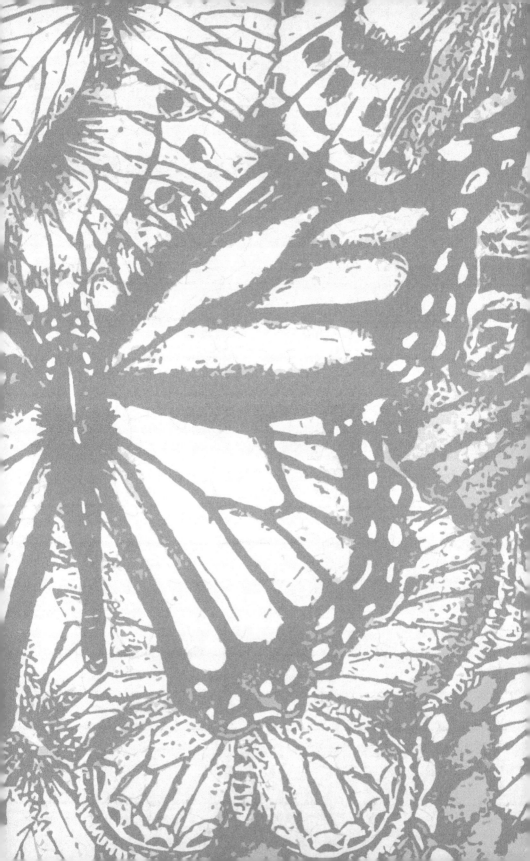

Maintaining Your Connections and Asking for Help

As a caregiver, you may feel overwhelmed by the ongoing problems, uncertainties, and changes brought on by dementia. It is easy to become lonely, believing you are alone in your troubles. On the other hand, maintaining connections and requesting help is valuable and necessary for your well-being as a caregiver.

Many carers struggle with the desire to bear the weight alone, believing they should be able to handle all the obstacles independently. However, this perspective frequently leads to burnout, exhaustion, and a decline in their mental and physical health. Maintaining connections allows you to build a network of people who can provide emotional support, practical aid, and a listening ear when you need it the most.

Reaching out to family members and friends or joining support groups for carers of loved ones with dementia can help you build and sustain connections. People who have faced similar challenges, can provide a solid foundation of empathy and understanding. Sharing your feelings, concerns, and frustrations with others who understand can help you feel less isolated and provide a safe environment for emotional release.

Asking for assistance is an unavoidable part of caregiving, yet it is frequently one of the most challenging steps. Caregivers often worry about burdening others with their duties. However, it is critical to understand that asking for help is not a show of weakness but rather a brave act of self-care. By reaching out, you allow others to assist you, share the burden, and provide respite, allowing you to continue providing the finest care for your loved one.

Remember that your well-being as a caregiver is as vital as caring for your loved one. By cultivating your support network, you establish a safety net that not only helps you negotiate the obstacles of dementia care but also enables you to provide your loved one with the ongoing support they require.

Reflect on your current support system. Who can you rely on for emotional support and assistance in your caregiving journey?

What barriers or hesitations do you have in asking for help? How can you overcome these obstacles and reach out to others?

How can you prioritize and actively maintain connections with friends and family while balancing your caregiving responsibilities?

Describe a time when you asked for help and received the support you needed. How did it impact your overall well-being and ability to care for your loved one?

Brainstorm creative ways to stay connected with loved ones and friends, mainly when time and energy are limited due to caregiving responsibilities.

How can you create a support network that understands and empathizes with your unique experiences as a dementia caregiver?

Explore the role of support groups and caregiver communities in maintaining connections and finding understanding. Have you ever participated in a support group or sought out a caregiver community? How did it impact your caregiving experience? If not, what are some steps you can take to connect with others who are going through similar challenges?

Reflect on the potential guilt or shame associated with asking for help when caring for a loved one with dementia. How can you modify your thoughts and let go of these negative emotions to embrace the support that is available to you?

Explore the concept of setting boundaries and learning to delegate tasks when caring for a loved one with dementia. How can you modify your thoughts and overcome any resistance to assigning responsibilities to others? How can you communicate your needs effectively and maintain a healthy balance as a caregiver?

Reflect on a time when you received help or support from someone unexpected. How did this experience impact your caregiving journey? How can you modify your thoughts to be more open and receptive to assistance from various sources?

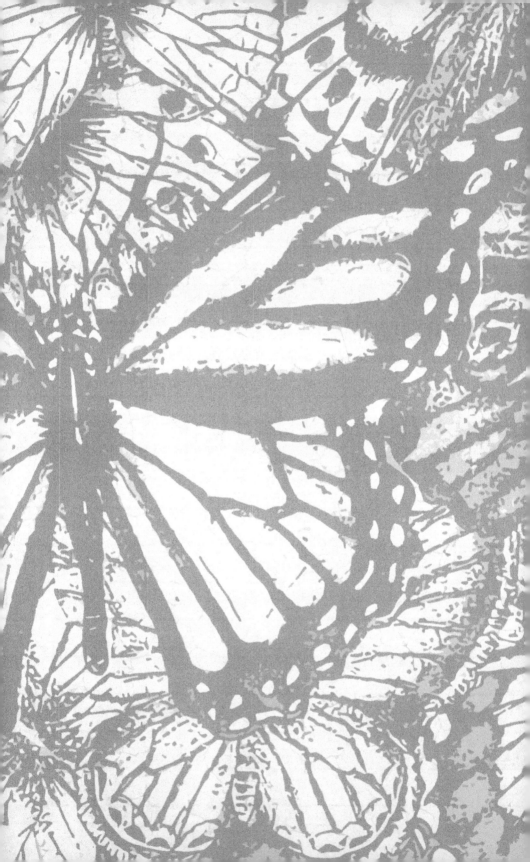

Caring for Your Own Body

It's tempting to put the needs of someone with dementia ahead of your own as a caretaker. However, it's critical to remember that caring for your body is just as vital. Your physical health directly impacts your ability to help your loved one. Consider your self-care routine and how well you've been treating your body. Consider the aspects of your physical health that you may have overlooked. Have you been getting enough sleep, eating good foods, and exercising regularly?

Consider tactics you might use to prioritize your physical health. Can you maintain a regular sleep routine or add healthier food options to your meals? Investigate other activities that interest you, such as walking, yoga, or dance.

Consider the significance of stress management in sustaining your physical health. Caring for someone with dementia is emotionally draining, and continuous stress can harm your health. Consider any symptoms of caregiver burnout you may have been feeling, such as tension, headaches, or fatigue.

Finally, explore several stress-reduction tactics you might implement in your everyday practice. Aside from medication, mindfulness activities, and prayer, indulging in hobbies or activities that offer you joy might help you reduce stress. Start thinking about how you may apply these ideas to your daily life.

Remember that caring for your body is not selfish. Prioritizing your well-being will better enable you to watch for the needs of your loved one. Acknowledge self-care as essential to your caregiving journey and prioritize your physical wellness.

Reflect on the physical toll that caregiving for someone with dementia can have on your body. How have you noticed your physical health being impacted? What steps can you take to prioritize self-care and ensure that you are taking care of your body while caring for your loved one?

Reflect on your current self-care routine. What are some physical activities or practices that bring you joy and help you stay physically healthy?

How can you prioritize regular exercise, even with the demands of caregiving? Brainstorm practical solutions and strategies.

How can you incorporate healthy eating habits into your daily routine, despite the challenges of caregiving? Share some simple, nourishing meal ideas.

What are some relaxation techniques, rituals, or hobbies that you can incorporate into your daily life to help alleviate stress and tension in your body?

Reflect on your current self-care routine. How well are you taking care of your physical health? Are there any areas where you can improve, such as regular exercise, eating a balanced diet, or getting enough sleep? What steps can you take to prioritize your physical well-being as a caregiver?

Reflect on your sleep patterns and the impact of caregiving on your quality of sleep. How can you modify your routine and establish a healthy sleep routine that allows you to prioritize rest and rejuvenation? What strategies or adjustments can you implement to improve the quality and quantity of your sleep?

Write about a specific self-care activity or practice that you find rejuvenating and helpful in caring for your body. How can you incorporate this activity into your regular routine? How does engaging in this activity improve your overall well-being?

Explore the concept of setting boundaries and establishing a support system to help you care for your body while caregiving. How can you communicate your needs to others, seeking their assistance or support? What resources or individuals can you rely on to help you maintain your physical health?

Reflect on the importance of self-compassion and forgiveness when it comes to taking care of your body while caring for someone with dementia. How can you modify your thoughts and release any guilt or judgment you may have towards yourself for prioritizing your own well-being? How can self-compassion positively impact your physical health and caregiving journey?

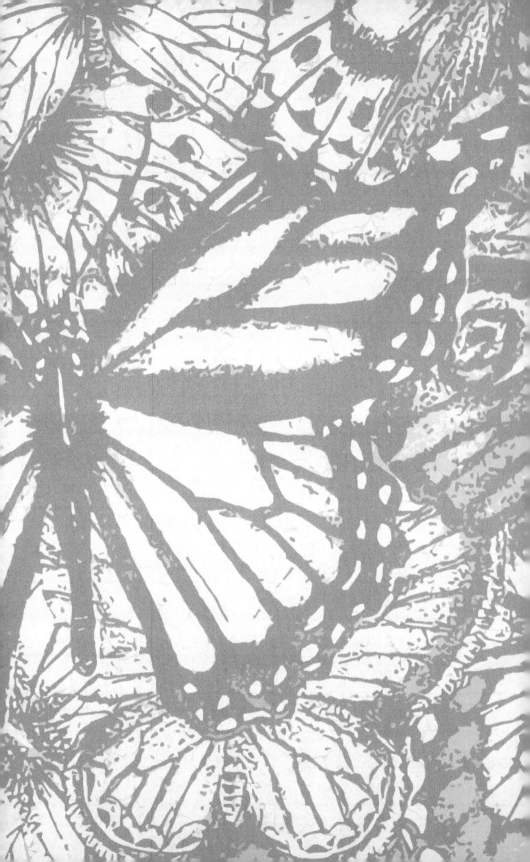

Taking Breaks

It's easy to get caught up in the demands of everyday activities as a caregiver for someone with dementia and forget to take time for yourself. Taking regular breaks, however, is critical for your health and capacity to give adequate care. Consider your routine and how you may add frequent breaks to your care plan.

Begin by selecting hobbies that bring you joy and allow you to unwind. These can be as easy as reading a book, going for a walk, indulging in a pastime, or practicing some mindfulness practices discussed in this journal. Make a list of activities you can do when taking a break.

Consider the resources and assistance available to aid in the facilitation of daily breaks. Is there a family member, friend, or neighbor who could help you with caregiving duties briefly? Are there respite care services available in the area to provide temporary relief? Investigate these alternatives and establish a list of any prospective sources of assistance.

Consider any obstacles that may impede your ability to take daily breaks. Are you feeling guilty or overwhelmed by the prospect of relinquishing your caring responsibilities? Consider these obstacles and remind yourself that taking breaks is not selfish but vital for your well-being.

Taking daily breaks is not a luxury but an essential element of being a competent caregiver. Commit to taking regular breaks from your caregiving duties. Set aside particular periods when you can get away from your caregiving responsibilities. Remember that by taking care of yourself, you are ensuring that you can continue to give your loved one the finest care possible.

How often do you take daily breaks to recharge and rejuvenate? Reflect on the impact these breaks have on your overall well-being.

Describe a recent situation where you felt overwhelmed and needed a break. How did you prioritize and make time for yourself in that moment?

Write about a specific activity or hobby that you enjoy and can engage in during your breaks. How can you modify your caretaking schedule and make a commitment to incorporate this activity into your regular break routine? How does engaging in this activity enhance your well-being and recharge your energy?

Reflect on the potential long-term consequences of neglecting to take breaks as a caregiver. How can you modify your thoughts and understand that by prioritizing your own needs, you are actually enhancing your ability to provide consistent and compassionate care? What strategies or systems can you put in place to ensure that you regularly take breaks?

Explore any guilt or resistance towards taking breaks as a caregiver. How can you reframe your mindset to view breaks as essential for your own well-being and the quality of care you provide?

How can you communicate your need for breaks to others involved in the caregiving process, such as family members or healthcare professionals? Brainstorm strategies for effective communication.

Reflect on a time when you prioritized and took a meaningful break. How did it positively impact your mental and emotional state, as well as your ability to care for your loved one?

Reflect on the impact of burnout and exhaustion on your ability to provide quality care. How can you modify your thoughts and recognize the importance of taking breaks as a means of preventing burnout? What strategies or boundaries can you establish to ensure that you regularly take necessary breaks for your own well-being?

Write about the fears or concerns you have about leaving your loved one with dementia while taking a break. How can you modify your thoughts and build a support system that allows you to feel confident and secure in taking breaks?

Explore the concept of respite care and it's benefits in providing temporary relief for caregivers. How can you seek respite care options that align with your needs and preferences? What steps can you take to research and explore respite care services available in your area?

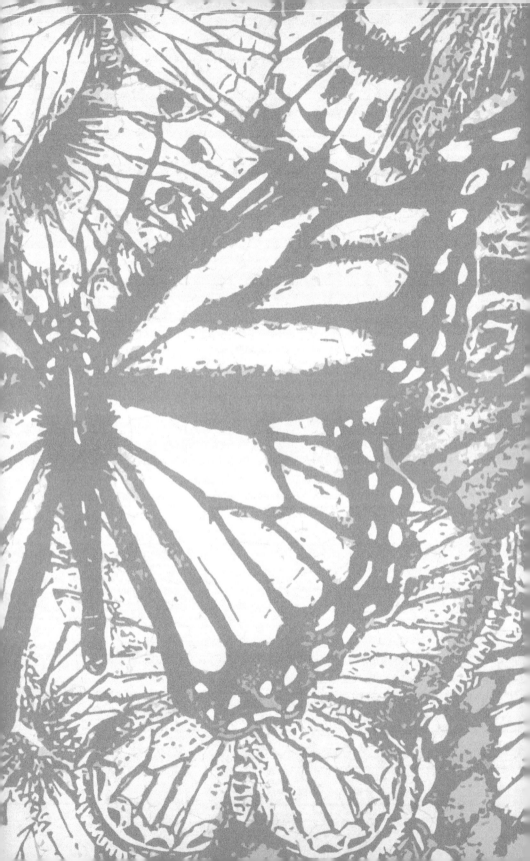

Processing Your Grief

Caring for someone with dementia can be emotionally taxing, and it's critical to recognize and handle the loss that comes with the situation. Allow yourself to experience and express your feelings of grief and sadness. Take some time to reflect on your caring experiences and emotions, and use this journal section to explore your grief.

Begin by recognizing the losses you have suffered as a caregiver. These losses could include the loss of the person your loved one once was, the loss of shared memories, or the loss of the future you had imagined together. Allow yourself to acknowledge your loss and validate your feelings honestly.

Consider how these losses have affected you emotionally. Are you experiencing sadness, anger, guilt, or a combination of these emotions? Taking the time to identify these feelings might help you better understand and process your grief.

Consider how you have dealt with the grief thus far. Have you given yourself time to grieve or suppressed your emotions? Consider the efficiency of the coping methods you've been practicing. If you haven't addressed your grief, consider how you may better assist yourself during this challenging period.

As a caregiver, allowing yourself the space and time to process your grief is essential. Talking to a trusted friend or family member, joining a support group, or seeking therapy are all options. Consider any resources or support systems you believe may be helpful. Remember that by identifying and processing your feelings, you can find healing and strength while continuing to care for your loved one.

Reflect on your current emotional state regarding your loved one's dementia diagnosis. How has it impacted your grief process and emotional well-being?

Describe a recent moment when you felt a wave of grief or sadness.
How did you cope with these emotions in that moment?

What are some healthy coping mechanisms or activities that can help you process your grief? How can you incorporate these into your daily routine?

How can you create a safe space for yourself to express and process your emotions surrounding your loved one's dementia? Consider journaling, therapy, or support groups as potential outlets.

Reflect on unresolved emotions or unfinished conversations with your loved one. How can you find closure or seek resolution in these areas?

Share a memory or experience that brings you comfort and joy amidst grief. How can you hold onto and cherish these moments as you navigate the caregiving journey?

Explore the impact of anticipatory grief on your well-being as a caregiver for someone with dementia. How does the gradual decline and loss of your loved one's cognitive abilities affect your emotional state? How can you navigate this complex form of grief while still providing the care and support they need?

Reflect on the role of acceptance in the grieving process when caring for a loved one with dementia. How can you find a balance between accepting the reality of their condition and allowing yourself to mourn the loss of their former self? What strategies or mindset shifts can you implement to help you come to terms with the changes and find peace amidst the grief?

Explore the potential conflicts and guilt that can arise when grieving while caring for a loved one with dementia. How do feelings of sadness or frustration intersect with the responsibility of providing care? How can you navigate these complex emotions and find ways to honor your own grief while still being present and supportive as a caregiver?

Reflect on the importance of finding meaning and purpose in your caregiving journey while processing grief. How can you find solace or a sense of fulfillment in the midst of sadness and loss? Are there any rituals, activities, or moments of connection with your loved one that bring you comfort or help you find a sense of purpose in your role as a caregiver?

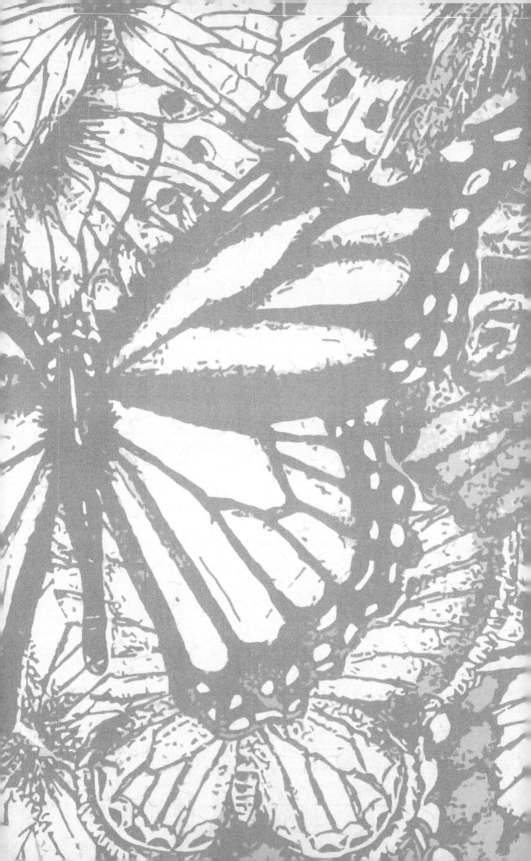

Cherishing the Memories Being Made

Caring for a loved one with dementia is a continual reminder of the fading memories. Despite the difficulties, there are still possibilities to make new memories and embrace the present. Reflect on the brief moments when new memories are made and acknowledge their value in this journal section.

Begin by recalling recent memories of your loved one that made you happy or smile. It could be as simple as a hug or a shared laugh. Recall this experience fully, paying attention to the sights, sounds, and feelings you experienced. This practice helps you realize the beauty and significance of these small moments in your caring journey.

Take into account the activities or interests that your loved one still appreciates. Consider how you and your loved one may include some of these activities into your routine. Participating in familiar and fun activities will help you connect and build new positive memories for both of you.

Consider the importance of touch and physical affection. A genuine connection can be formed by holding hands, delivering a soft hug, or even brushing your loved one's hair. Consider a time when physical touch provided comfort or joy to your loved one and how it made you feel as a carer. Recognizing the importance of these small actions will help you appreciate them even more.

You can discover joy and contentment in your role as a caretaker by embracing the small moments when new memories are formed. These are fleeting moments, but their significance can have a long-term influence on you and your loved one because they demonstrate the love and connection that remains despite the challenges of dementia.

Reflect on a recent positive and meaningful moment you shared with your loved one despite their dementia. How did it make you feel, and how can you cherish that memory?

What are some creative ways to capture and preserve new memories with your loved one, given the challenges of dementia? Consider photography, writing, or other forms of artistic expression.

How can you shift your focus from dwelling on the loss of memories to embracing and cherishing the present moments with your loved one?

Explore any fears or anxieties about losing more memories as your loved one's dementia progresses. How can you find solace in knowing that you can create new memories together?

Describe a recent activity or outing you enjoyed with your loved one. How can you intentionally create more opportunities for these joyful experiences?

How can you involve other family members or friends in creating and cherishing new memories with your loved one? Brainstorm collaborative activities or traditions that can bring everyone closer together.

Consider the small, everyday moments that you and your loved one share. What are some simple activities or routines that you both enjoy? How can you find gratitude in these moments and cherish them as precious gifts, even if they may seem mundane or routine?

Explore the concept of finding beauty in the present moment, even amidst the challenges of caregiving. How can you cultivate a mindset of gratitude and appreciation for the new memories being made with your loved one? Are there any practices or strategies that help you stay present and fully engaged in these moments?

Reflect on the role of storytelling and reminiscing in cherishing the new memories being made. How can you preserve and pass down the stories and experiences of your loved one, even as their memory fades? Consider writing down or recording their stories, or sharing them with others who may benefit from hearing them.

Consider the bittersweet nature of cherishing new memories with your loved one, knowing that their dementia will continue to progress. How can you find a balance between acknowledging the sadness or loss that may come, while also fully embracing and cherishing the joy and love present in each new memory?

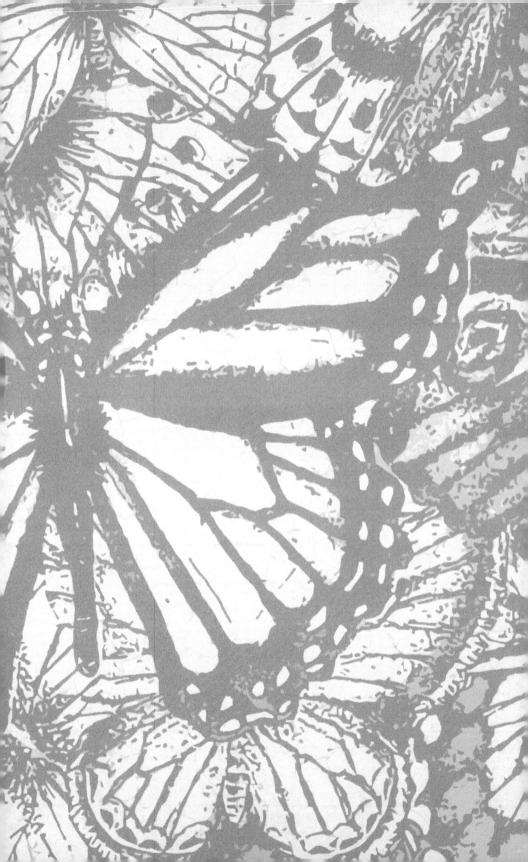

Final Thoughts

Resilience is the strength that enables us to overcome hardship, find hope in the face of despair, and persevere even when the road appears impossible. As caretakers, we've been tested in ways we never imagined, but we've also discovered an inner resilience we didn't know we had. We have discovered the ability to keep going and to find moments of joy amidst the chaos because of our resilience.

Dementia caregiving is more than just the physical activities we complete or our medical decisions. It is a journey of the heart, a profound human experience that pushes us to grow, expand, and discover new aspects of ourselves. This journey teaches us to appreciate the beauty in the minor details, such as the flickering light of recognition in our loved one's eyes, the gentle touch of their hand, or the sweet whisper of their voice.

We learn to seek meaning amid our caregiving journey. Even in the face of loss and decline, we uncover opportunities for connection, love, and transformation. We learn to discover significance not only in the life of our loved ones but also in our own lives by enjoying the present moment and finding purpose in our caregiving role. When our caregiving journey ends, we take the lessons we've learned, the strength we've gained, and the resilience we've developed. Ultimately, we find comfort in knowing that we did our best, that our love and care made a difference, and that, even in the face of "The Longest Goodbye," our path as caregivers was one of enormous meaning and purpose.

In loving memory of my mother, who's long battle with Frontotemporal Dementia could not steal her resilient and determined spirit. And to my father, whose selflessness and devotion in caring for her throughout her illness was an inspiring example of unconditional love and commitment.

About the Author

Kellie Vanella is an autistic self-advocate, mother, writer, and special education advocate. She resides in Virginia with her husband and three children.

To find more of Kellie's work, go to UnmaskAutism.com.

Made in the USA
Las Vegas, NV
22 March 2024

87617326R00118